Happy Birthday, Robert
March 29, 1977
Aunt Frances

What Happens at an Animal Hospital

by Arthur Shay

REILLY & LEE BOOKS · CHICAGO

This book is for Marlin Perkins, who explained to me, around a twilight campfire in Kenya, why he was devoting his life to animals: "They need us."

Copyright © 1972 by Arthur Shay. All rights reserved.
Published by Reilly & Lee Books, a division of Henry Regnery Company
114 West Illinois Street, Chicago, Illinois 60610
Library of Congress Catalog Card Number: 72-80956
International Standard Book Number: 0-8092-8608-4
Manufactured in the United States of America

To Parents and Teachers

If you've ever eavesdropped in elevators, skimmed through the "health" column of your local paper, or sat for very long at a desk in a large office, you must be aware that many humans are voluble hypochondriacs.

But what of the billions of other animals with whom we share our troubled planet? Of course, they suffer from illness and injury just as we do. But for the most part, they suffer in silence.

"The fact is," said Dr. Lloyd Prasuhn, the soft-voiced, skilled veterinarian I visited for this book, "that the inability of dogs and cats to tell you what's wrong with them is what got me interested in veterinary medicine way back around the Korean War. To me there is nothing more fulfilling than to help another creature in pain.

"Soon, though," he added, "I found that animals communicate all over the place. You just get to know the signs—the way they breathe, move, eat, and respond. Why, some of them tell you *more* than human patients! Sometimes, animals even *malinger,* just to be fussed over or to get out of the house and down here to the hospital for a vacation."

It's hard to blame this sort of wily creature. From the heavy-duty air filtration system that keeps the hospital odorless and relatively germ-free to the spotless cages, the modern animal hospital equals—and in many cases, unfortunately, surpasses—some human hospitals I've visited. There are recovery rooms, ECG machines, and even a brain-wave monitor to search a pet's cranium for abnormalities. To shoot the surgery sequence for this book, I had to gown-up and seal my camera's possible staph germs in plastic wrap!

It might be productive and even *fun* for parents or teachers using this book with young humans to have them mime the various symptoms of distress that animals can't describe for their doctors: "You're a dog with a bellyache . . ."

These improvisations might add a dimension to what I hope is a comprehensive visit to a modern animal hospital.

Arthur Shay

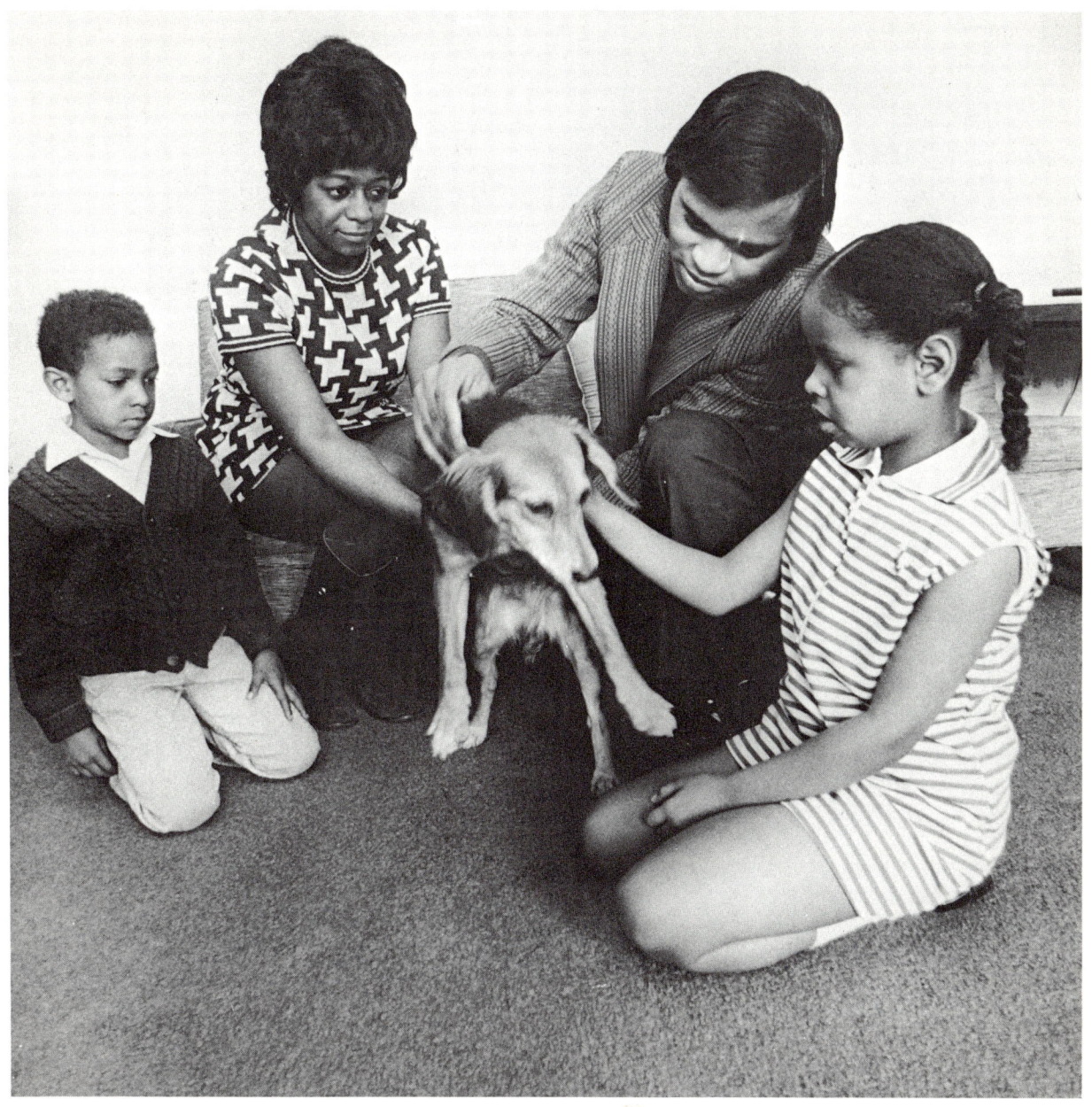

For nearly a week, the Reed family's dog, Bambi, hadn't been feeling well. "She's been coughing a lot," said Angie Reed to her father.

"Poor puppy," said Angie's mother, stroking Bambi's soft brown fur. "She doesn't seem to be eating well, either. She even turned down some liver today!"

Tony Reed said, "And Bambi has become so *lazy*. This morning she wouldn't run out to the ball field with me. She wouldn't even carry my glove!"

"Hmm," said Mr. Reed. "I think we'd better take Bambi to the animal hospital. She's due for a checkup anyway."

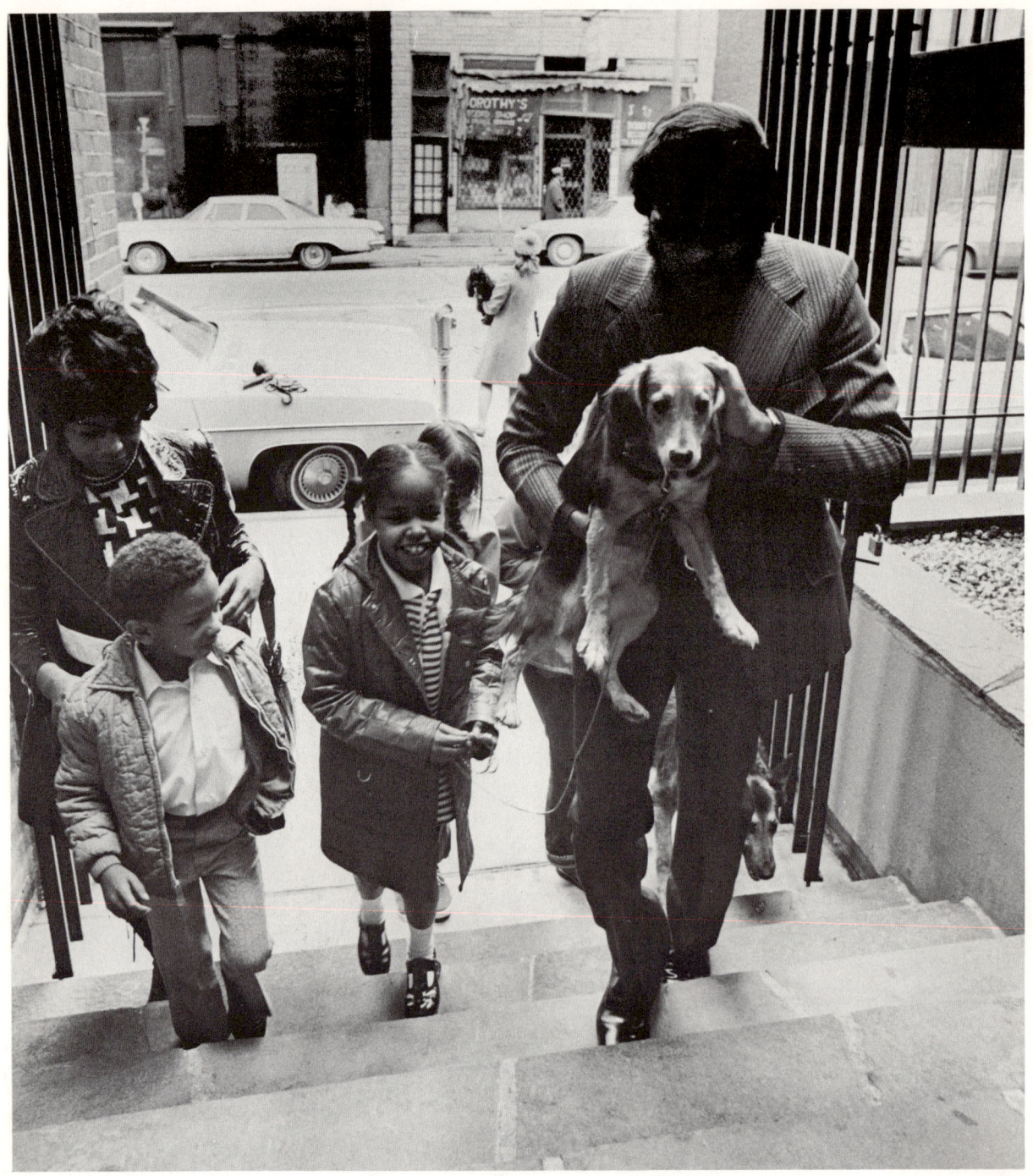

As usual, Bambi seemed to like the car ride. But she wasn't strong enough to climb the steps to the Lake Shore Animal Hospital in Chicago, so Mr. Reed carried her in.

The animal hospital is a busy place where animal doctors, or *veterinarians*, and other hospital workers, called *attendants*, care for dogs, cats, birds, and other animals. Lake Shore has just about the same equipment for taking care of animals that other hospitals have for helping sick humans.

The Reeds gave their name and Bambi's to the *receptionist* at the front desk.

"We'd like to see Dr. Prasuhn," said Ms. Reed. "He gave Bambi her first shots, so she'll recognize him and won't be too scared."

"Dr. Prasuhn will be here in a few minutes," said the receptionist. "He's in the emergency room right now."

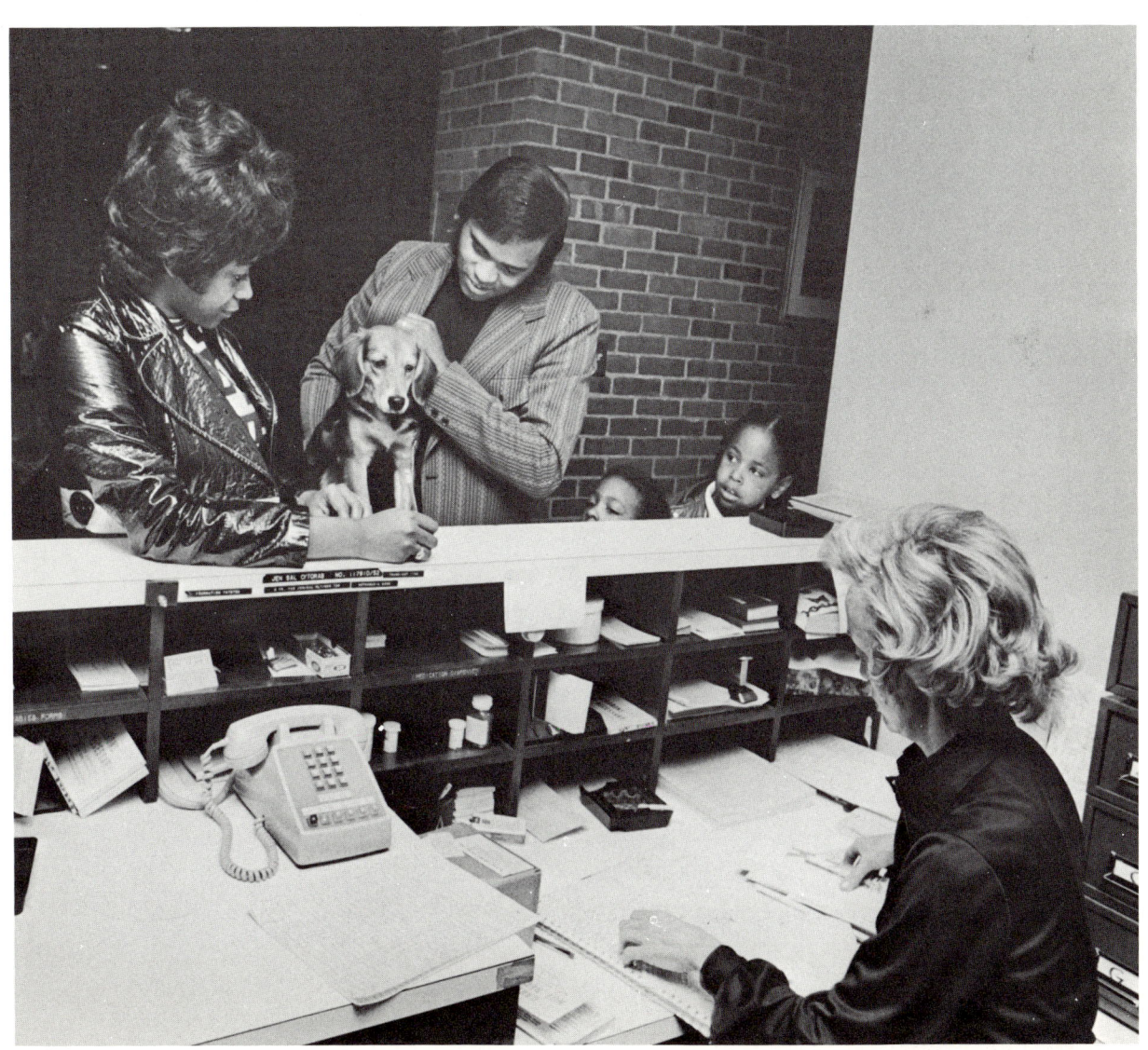

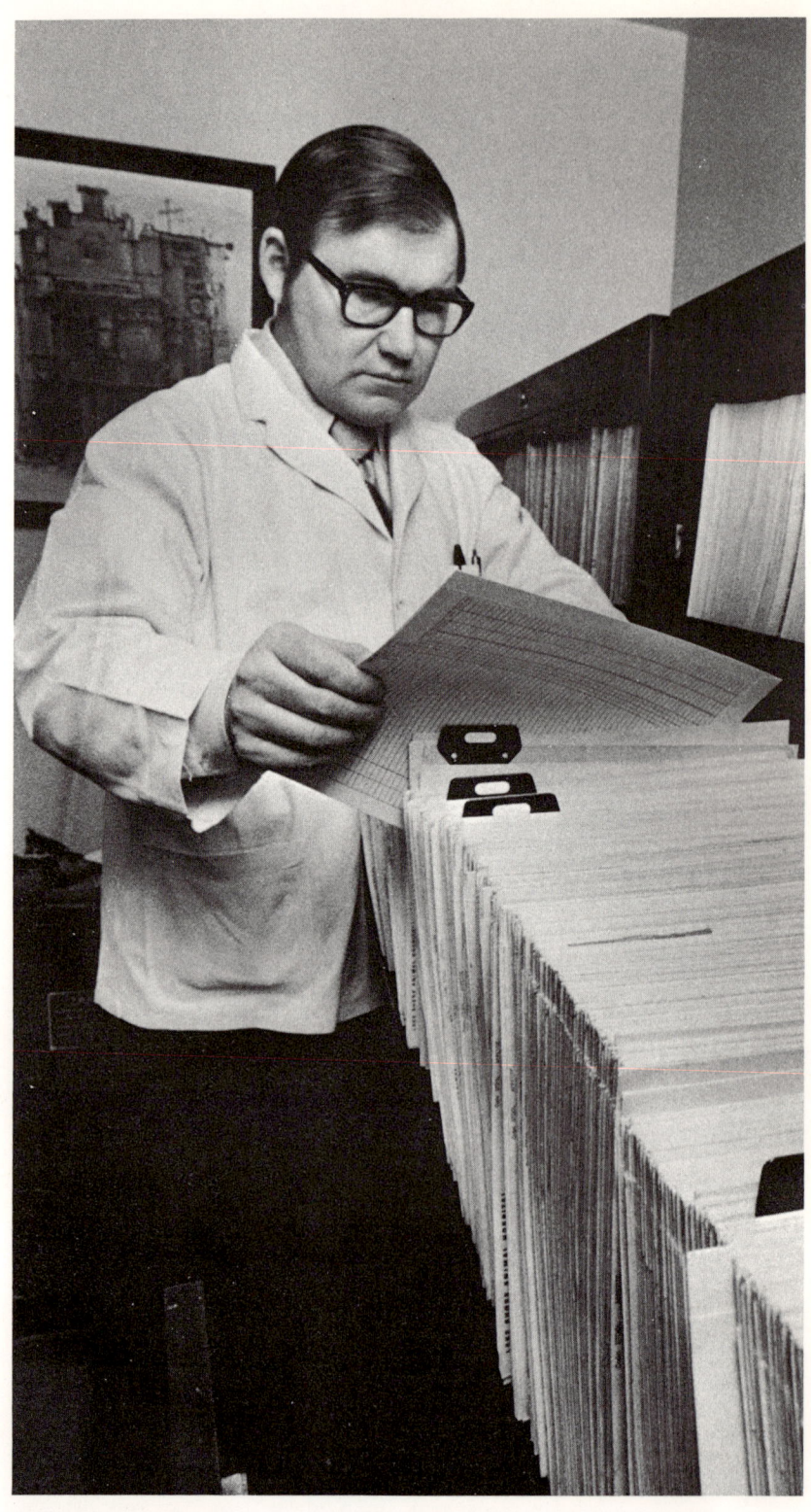

The first thing Dr. Lloyd Prasuhn did was to look at Bambi's medical record. Lake Shore Animal Hospital has a file folder for each of its patients. Bambi's record was filed under "R" for Reed.

While Mr. and Ms. Reed checked over Bambi's health record with the receptionist to make sure their pet's shots were up to date, Dr. Prasuhn invited Angie and Tony into an examining room. He looked into Bambi's eyes, ears, nose, and throat and felt around her neck to see if her glands were swollen.

"How has Bambi been behaving?" he asked the children.

"She hasn't eaten well for a week," said Angie sadly. "She coughs a lot—"

"And she's too lazy to carry my glove to the ball field," added Tony.

"I see," said Dr. Prasuhn. Then he listened to Bambi's heart with an instrument called a *stethoscope*.

"Hmm," was all he said.

"The doctor looks worried to me," Angie whispered to her younger brother. "I hope it's nothing serious."

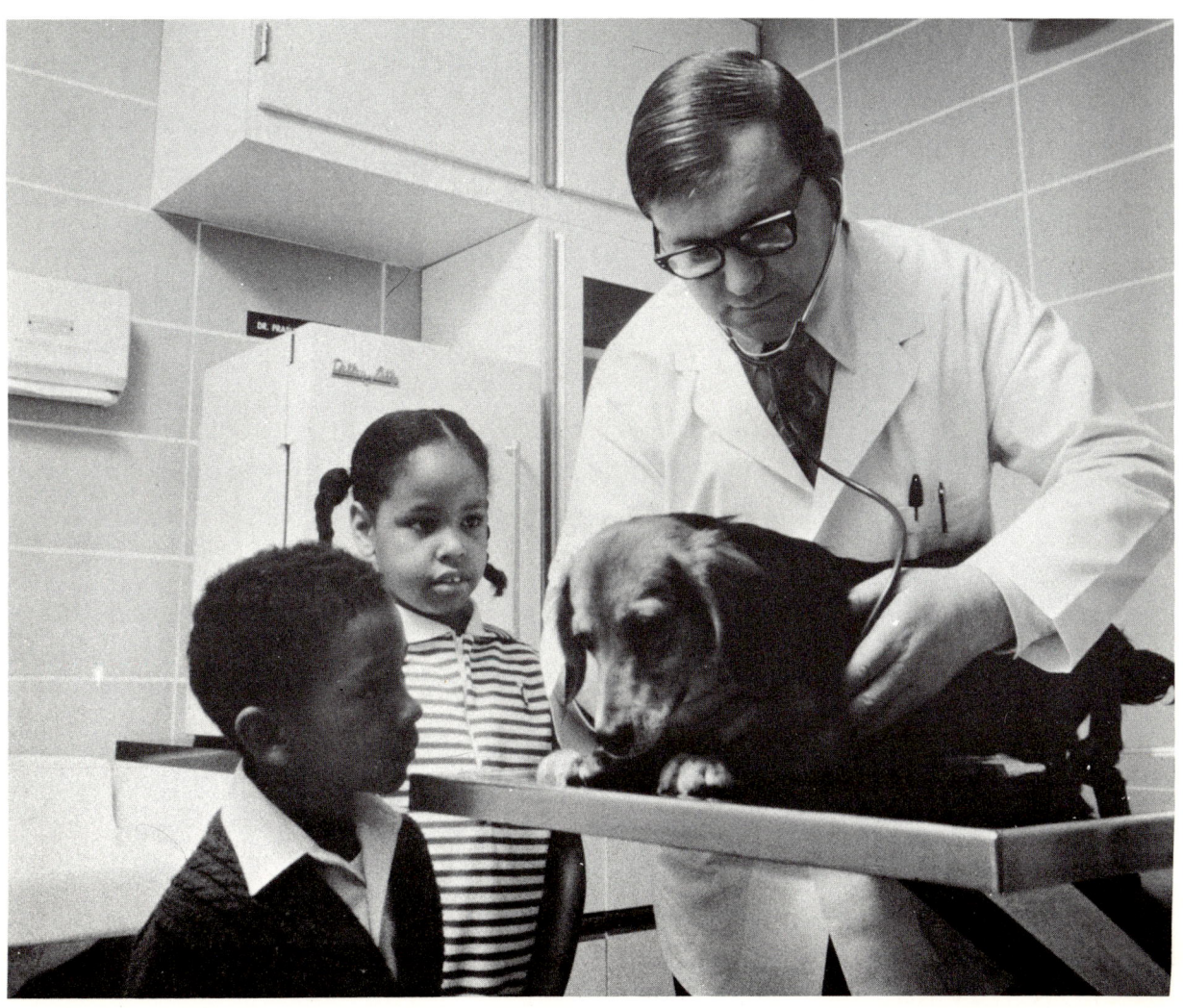

In the lobby, Dr. Prasuhn told the Reeds that he wanted to give Bambi a test called an ECG.

"We run it on a machine that's connected to the patient by wires. The machine tells us if the heart is pumping properly. Dr. Harris and my assistant, John Kampfer, are experts at running this test. It won't take long. And it doesn't hurt," the doctor said.

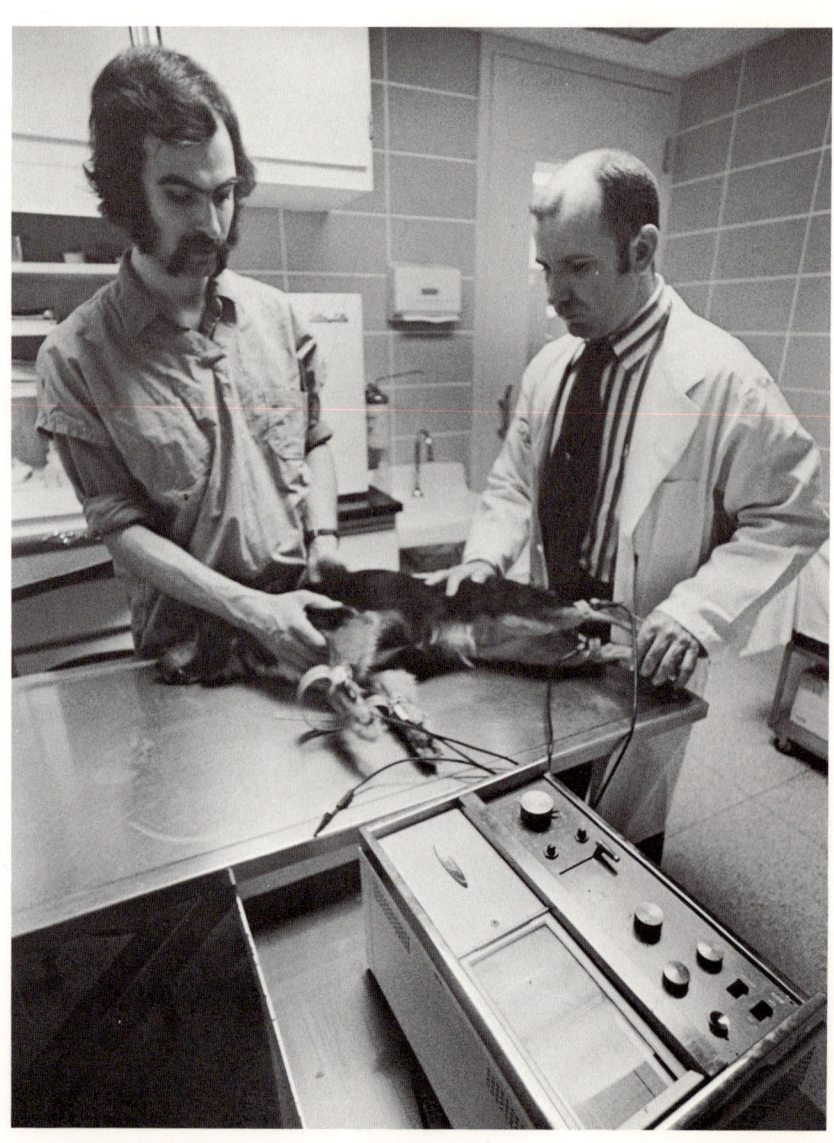

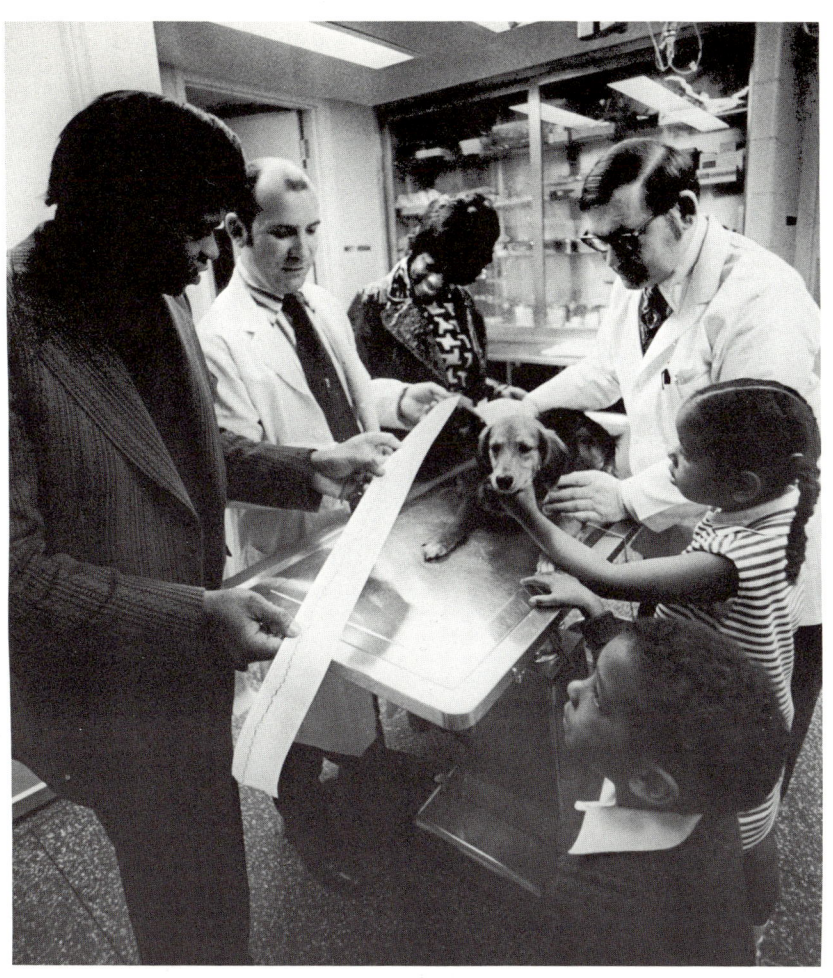

The ECG machine prints out a wiggly line that gives doctors a picture of how well the heart is doing its work. Dr. Prasuhn showed the Reeds the wiggly lines that Bambi's heart had made on a long roll of paper.

"What does it mean?" Angie asked with a frown.

"It means," said Dr. Prasuhn, "that Bambi has a little heart trouble."

"Uh-oh," said Tony. "That's bad."

"Not in Bambi's case, Tony," said Dr. Prasuhn. "Luckily, it's just a minor problem, nothing serious. It's called *patent ductus arteriosus* in Latin. The blood is not flowing normally through Bambi's heart. But I think we can fix her up with an operation."

The doctor looked at Angie and Tony. "Bambi will have to stay at the hospital for a few days," he said.

"Sounds good," said Mr. Reed. "We want a healthy pet."

Angie and Tony didn't look happy at all. Bambi had not spent a night away from home since she had come to live with the Reeds.

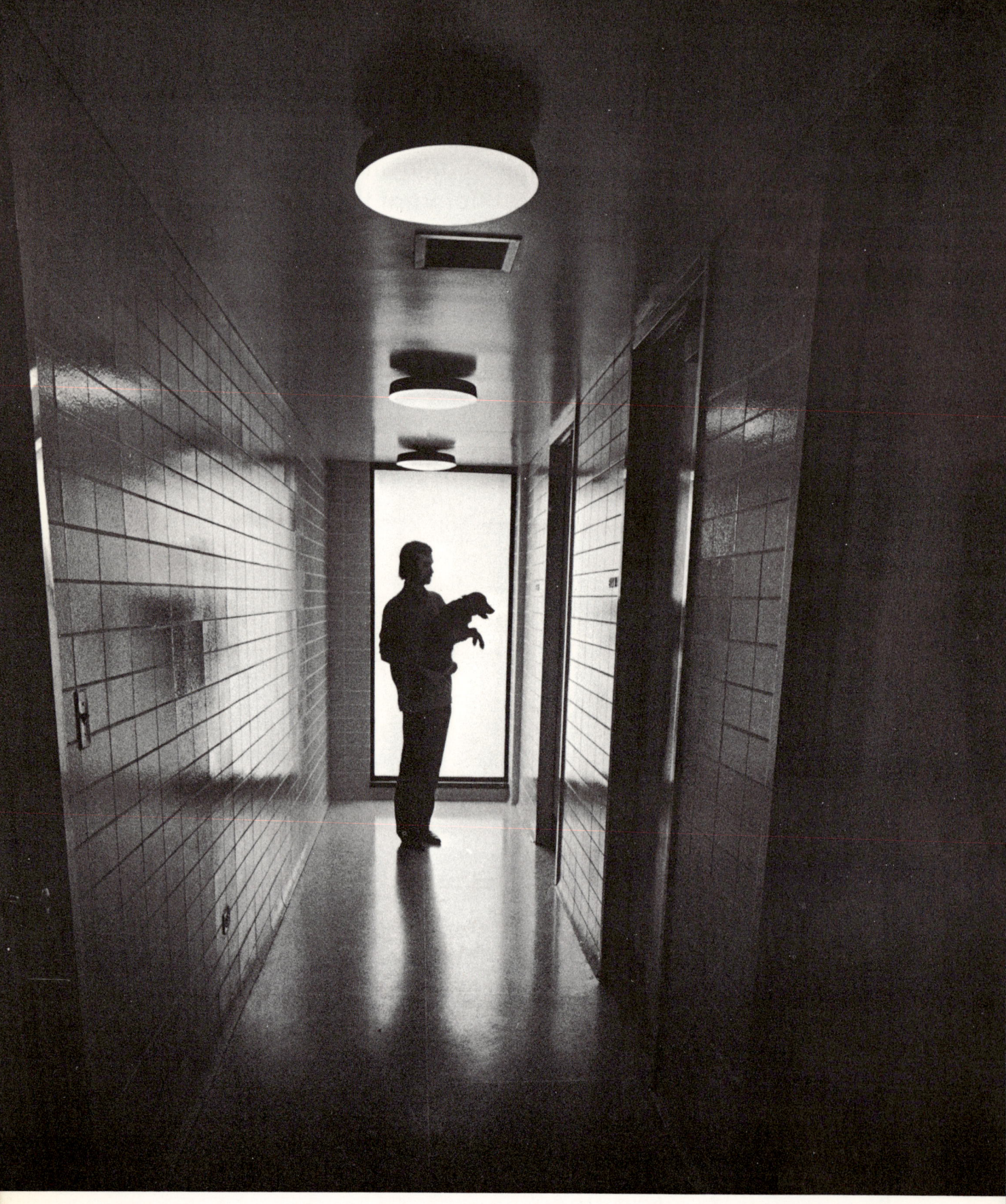

The children watched sadly as John carried Bambi down the long hospital corridor to the kennel area. "Don't worry," said the doctor as he left the Reeds. "Bambi will be just fine."

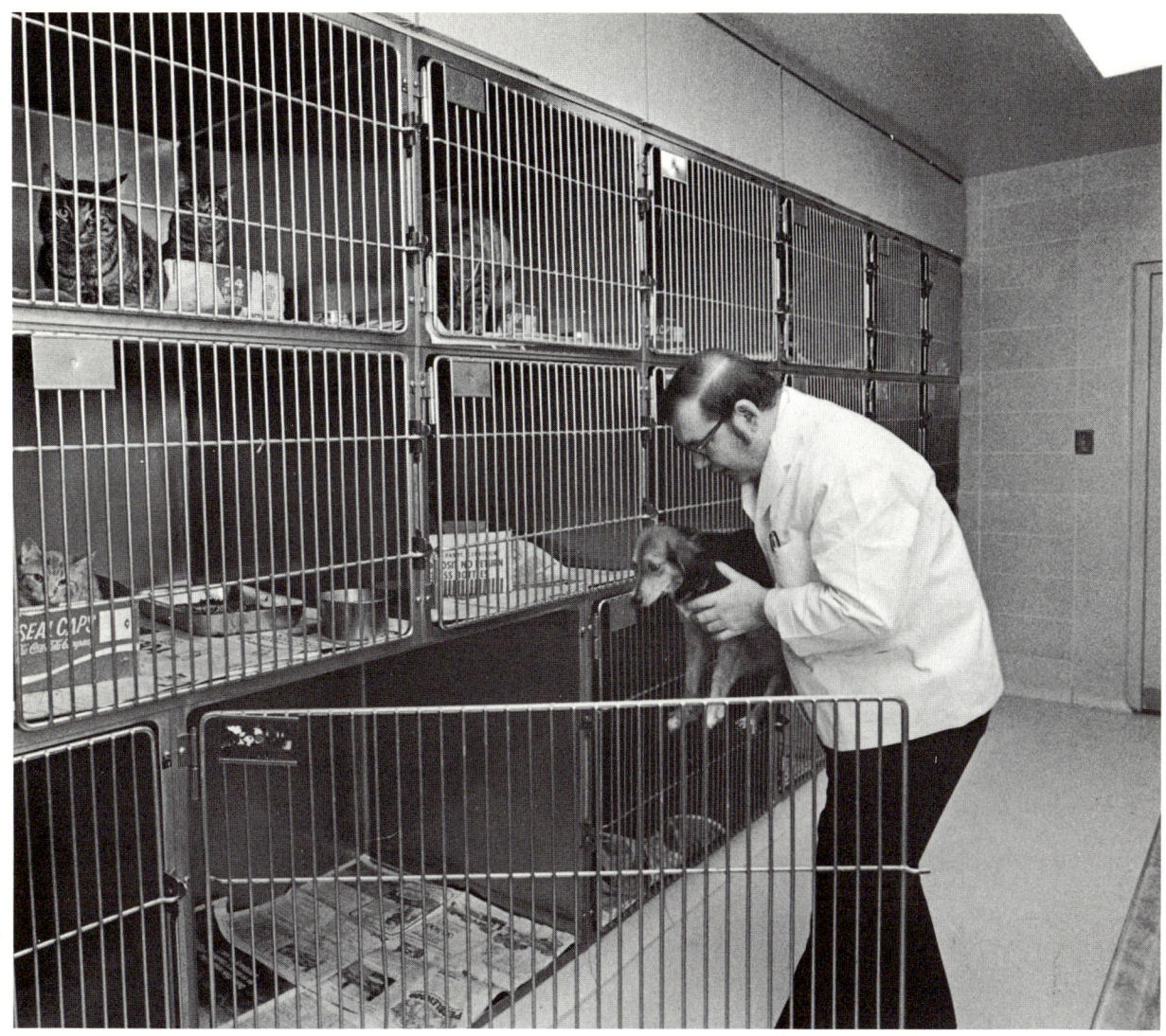

Dr. Prasuhn took Bambi from John and gently placed her into a kennel.

"You'll be staying here for a few days, Bambi," he said. "You'll need some time to heal after your operation."

Then the doctor patted her head and went back to talk with the Reeds.

Bambi found herself in a strange room with twenty dogs and cats she had never met before, and on top of that, she wasn't feeling too well. But she behaved like a good dog and didn't bark once.

Back with the Reeds, Dr. Prasuhn said, "If Bambi had a disease that was catching, we'd put her in the isolation ward. It has a separate air-conditioning and filtering system, which helps us keep germs from spreading."

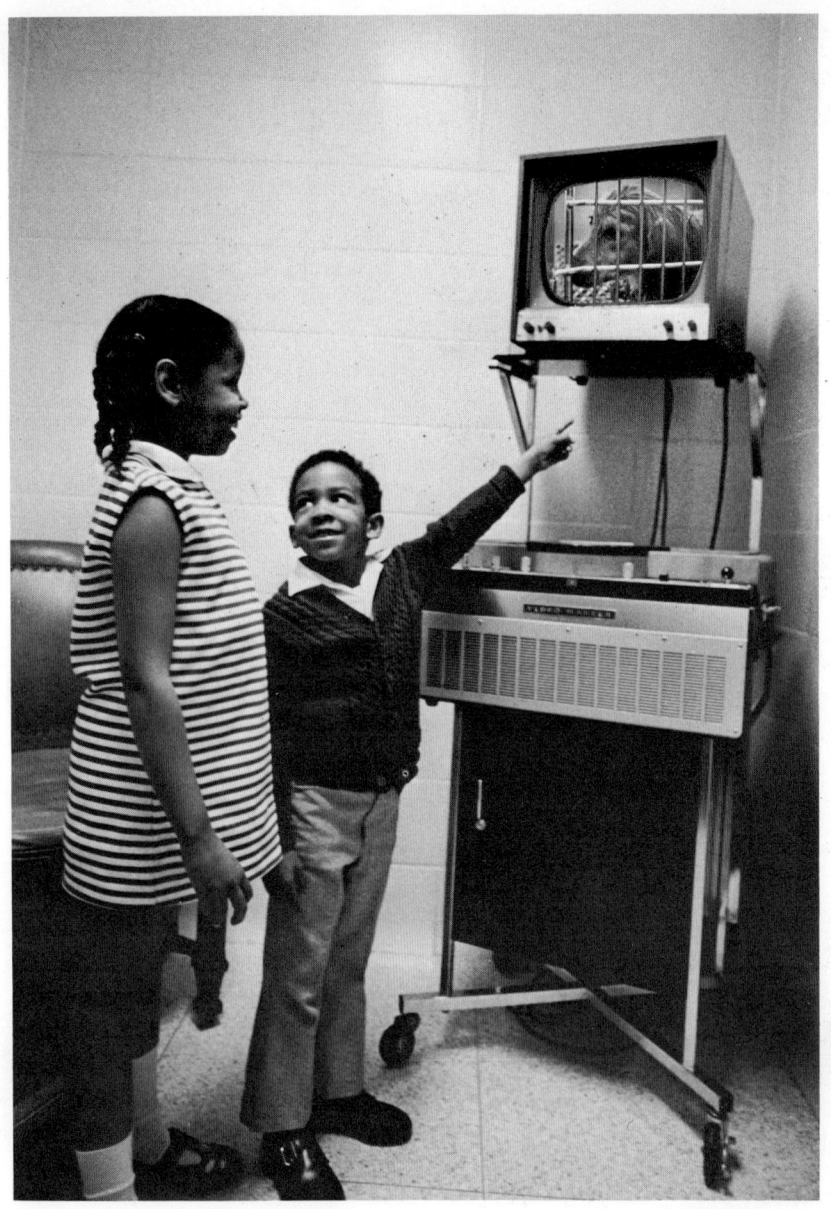

"I miss Bambi already, lazy or not," said Tony, holding back tears.

"When can we come to see her?" Angie asked.

"I can't let you visit Bambi in person," the doctor said. "It might disturb the other patients. But I can do the next best thing. I can let you see for yourself how Bambi's doing—on television."

"Wow!" said Ms. Reed as the doctor led them down another hallway. "Closed-circuit TV!"

"Yes, ma'am," said Dr. Prasuhn. "Okay, kids, you stay here in the viewing room. I'll go back and set up the camera."

Soon the Reeds were able to see Bambi on TV.

"She looks like she's in a dog food commercial," said Angie, laughing at last.

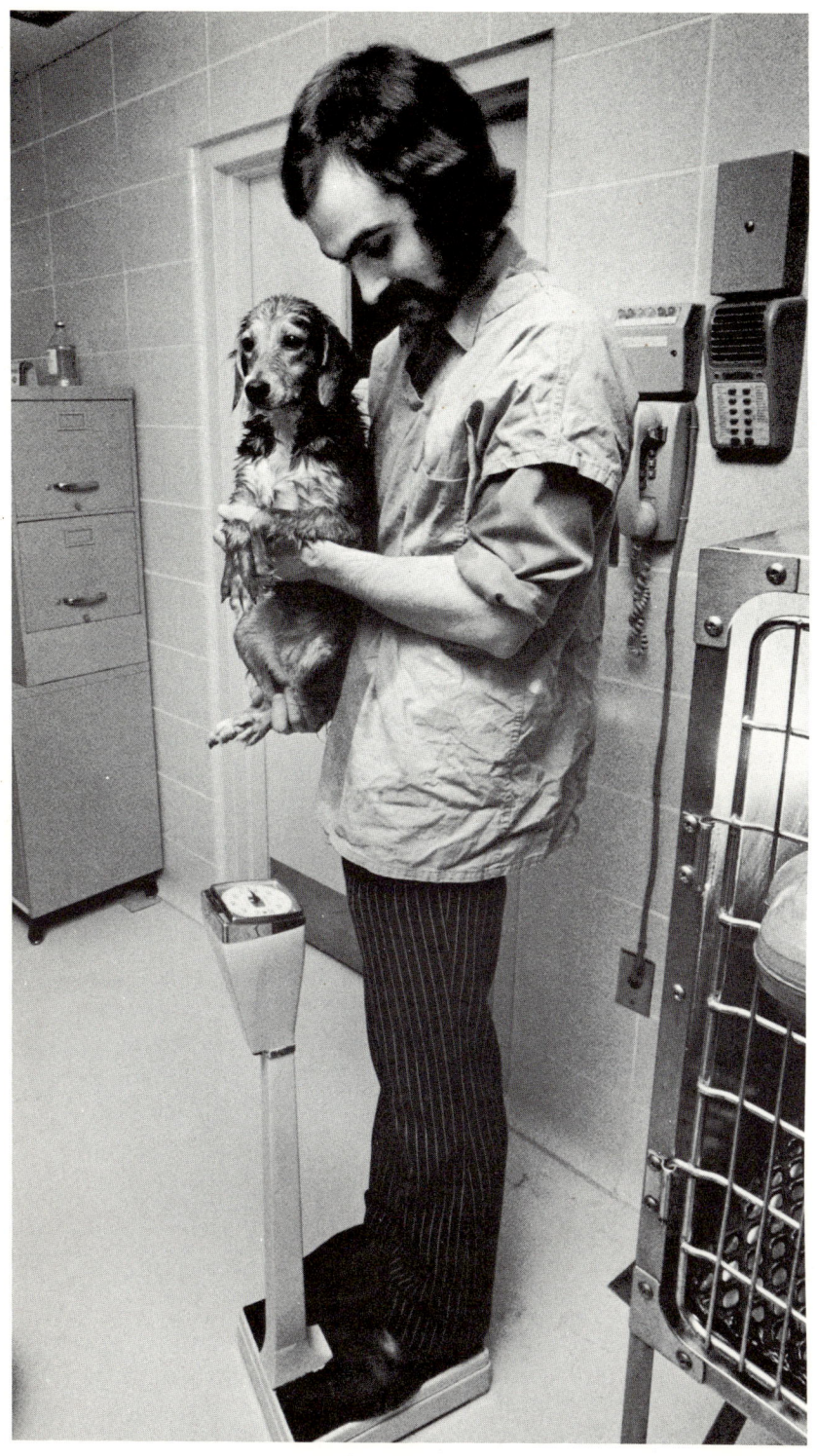

The next morning, John Kampfer, who is studying to be a veterinarian, was ready to guide Bambi through her first full day at the hospital. First he weighed her. The easy way to weigh dogs or cats is to weigh yourself, then take your pet onto the scale with you. John weighed 140 pounds alone. With Bambi in his arms he weighed 160. Can you figure out how much Bambi weighed?

"I don't mean to hurt your feelings, Bambi," said John, "but I have to give you your bath now."

At Lake Shore Animal Hospital, dogs are rinsed from the head backward to the tail, so that fleas and germs are washed away from the head. Bambi didn't like the high-pressure spray very much.

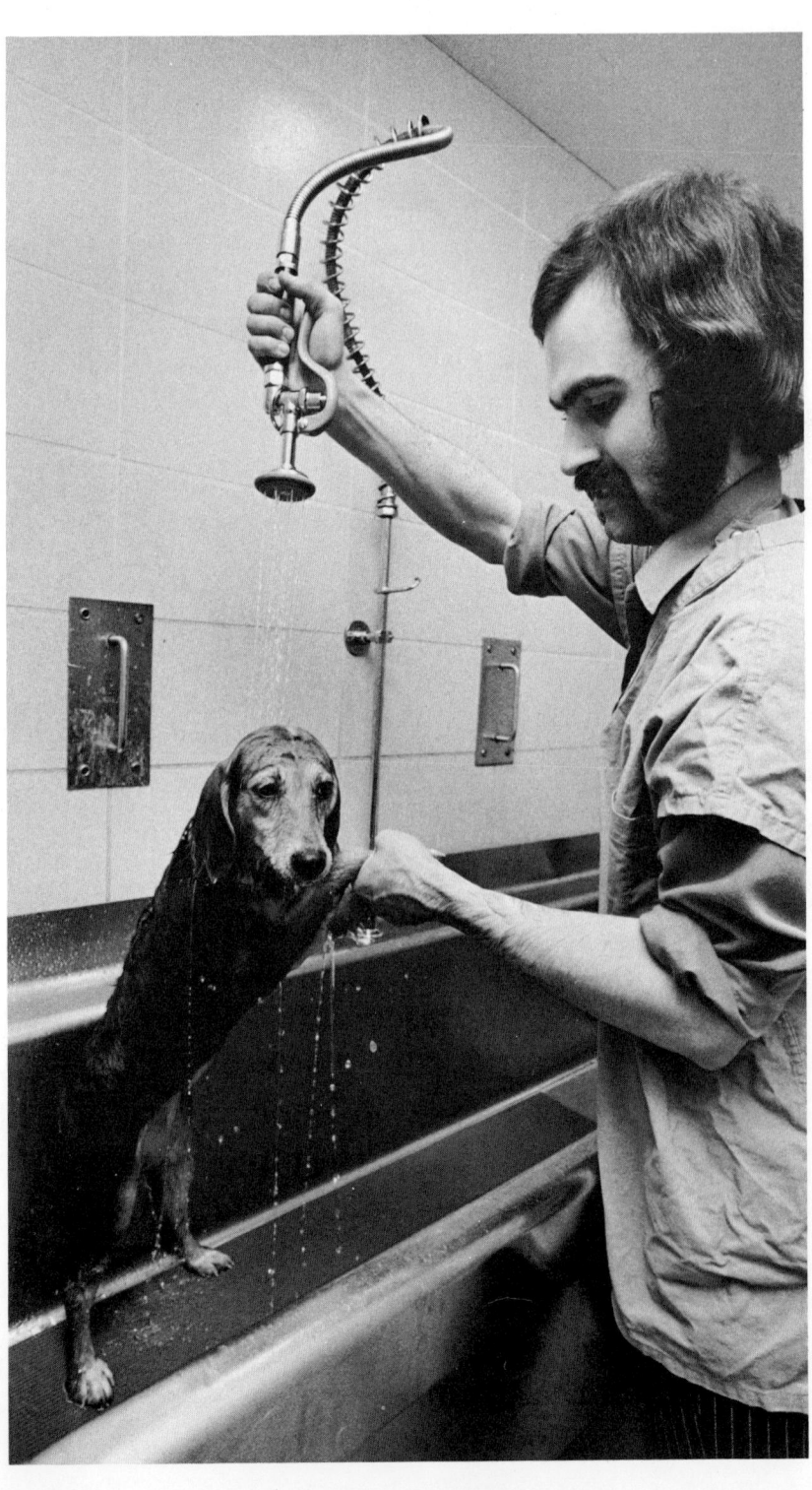

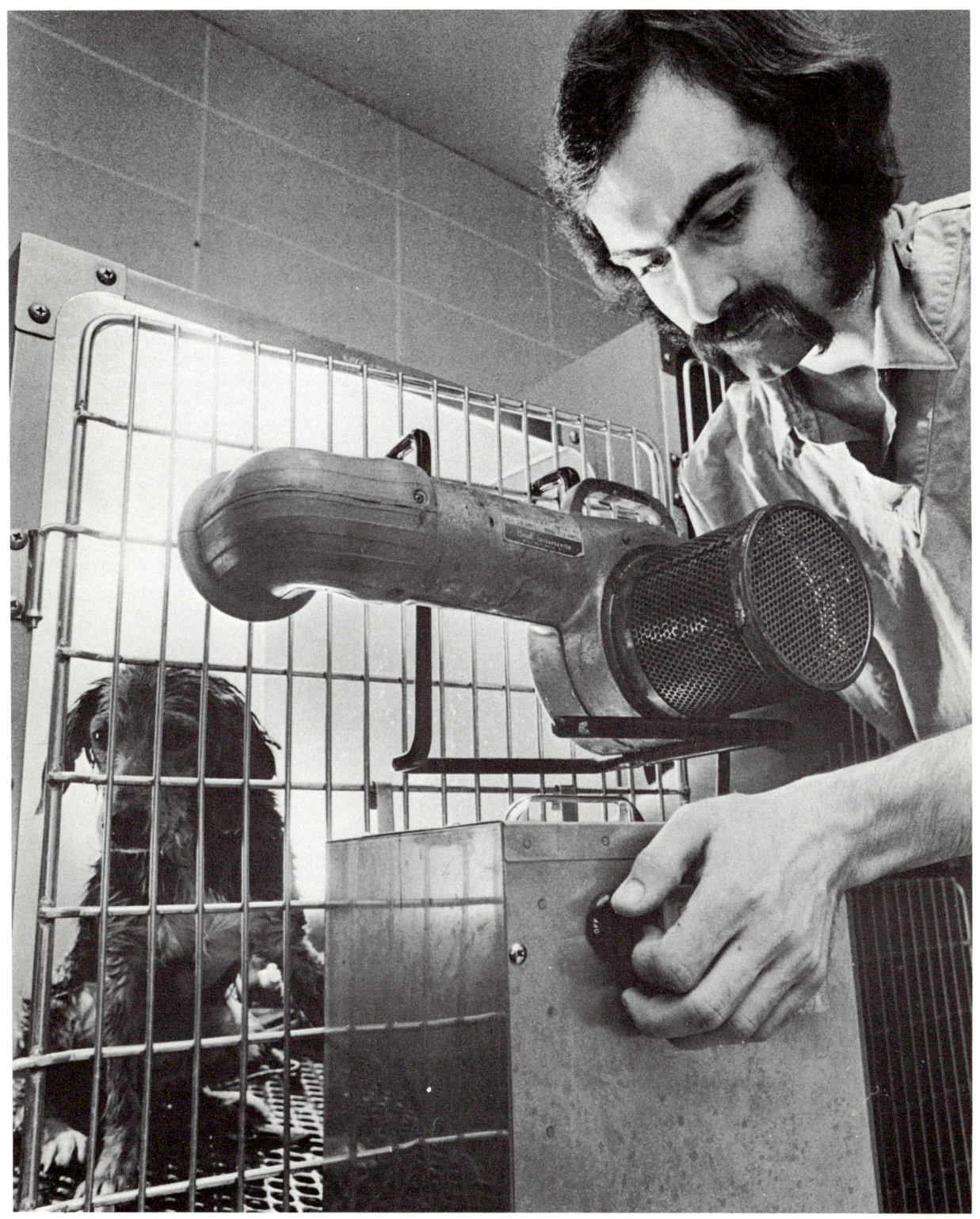

But in a few minutes she was enjoying herself under a hot-air dryer.

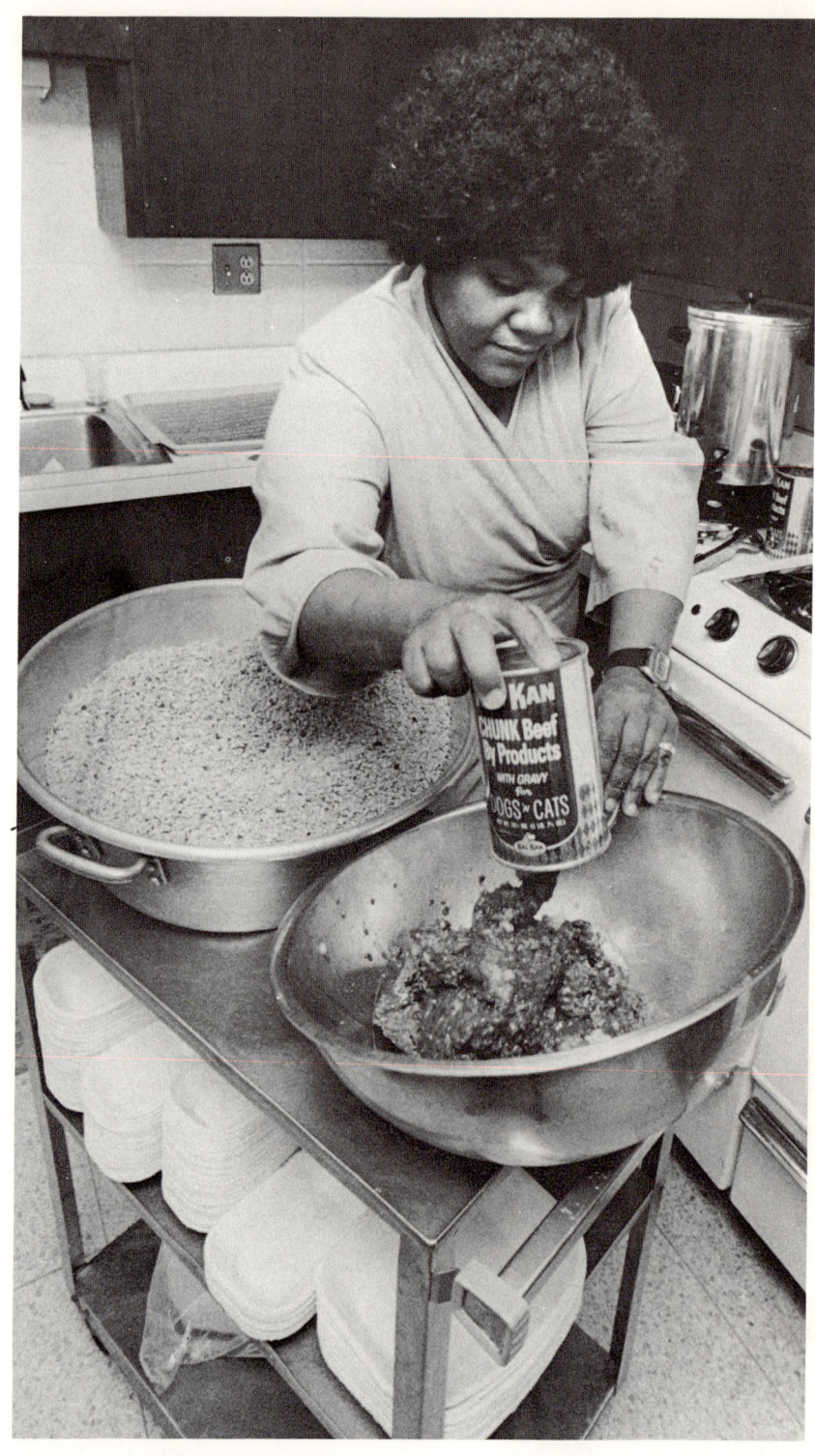

Meanwhile, another attendant was in the kitchen preparing food for the 250 patients at Lake Shore Animal Hospital. The animals are fed from this cart twice a day. You can see the paper plates under the big bowls of food.

"Here you are, Bambi," said the attendant who dropped off Bambi's meal. "I know you don't have much of an appetite, but please try to eat at least a little."

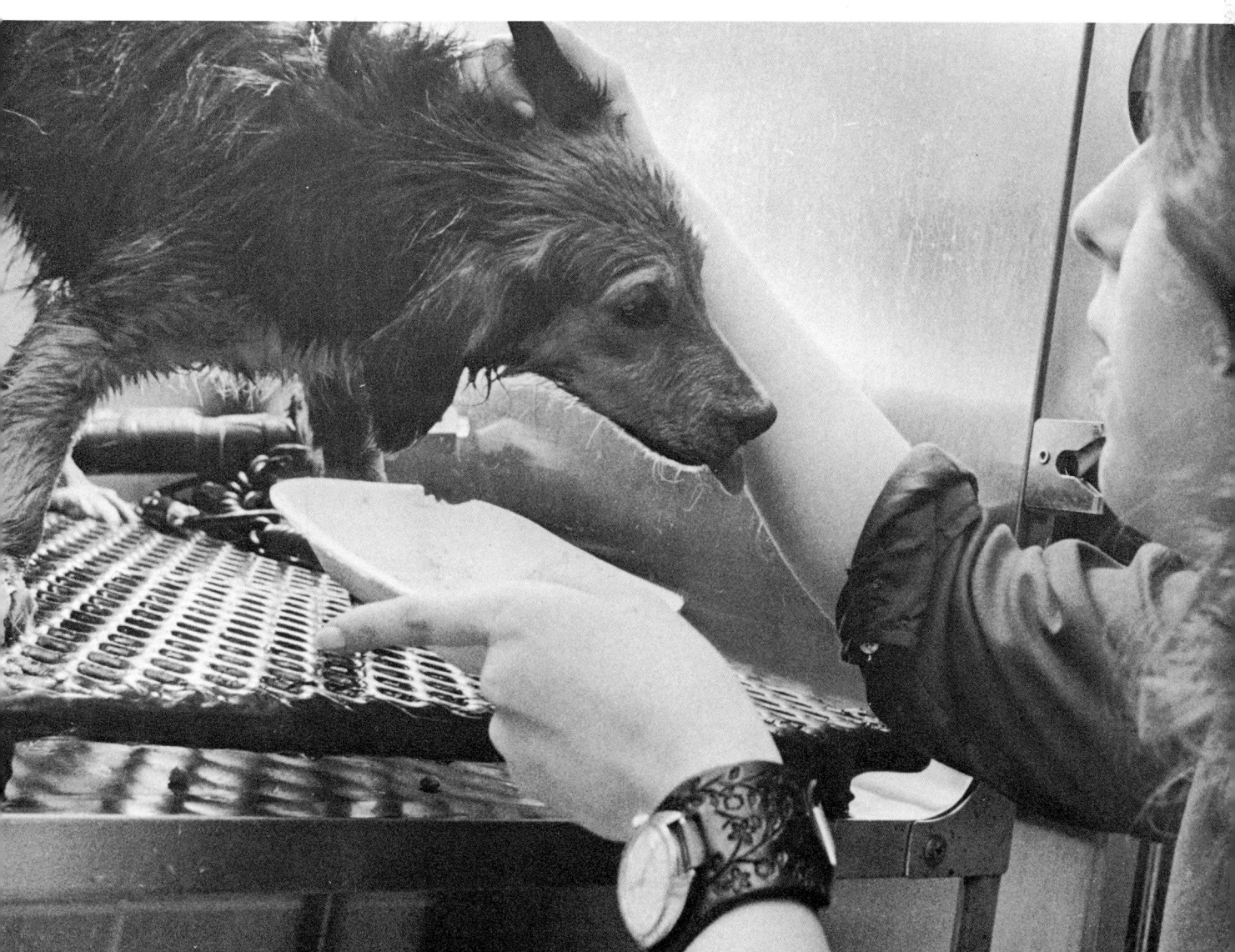

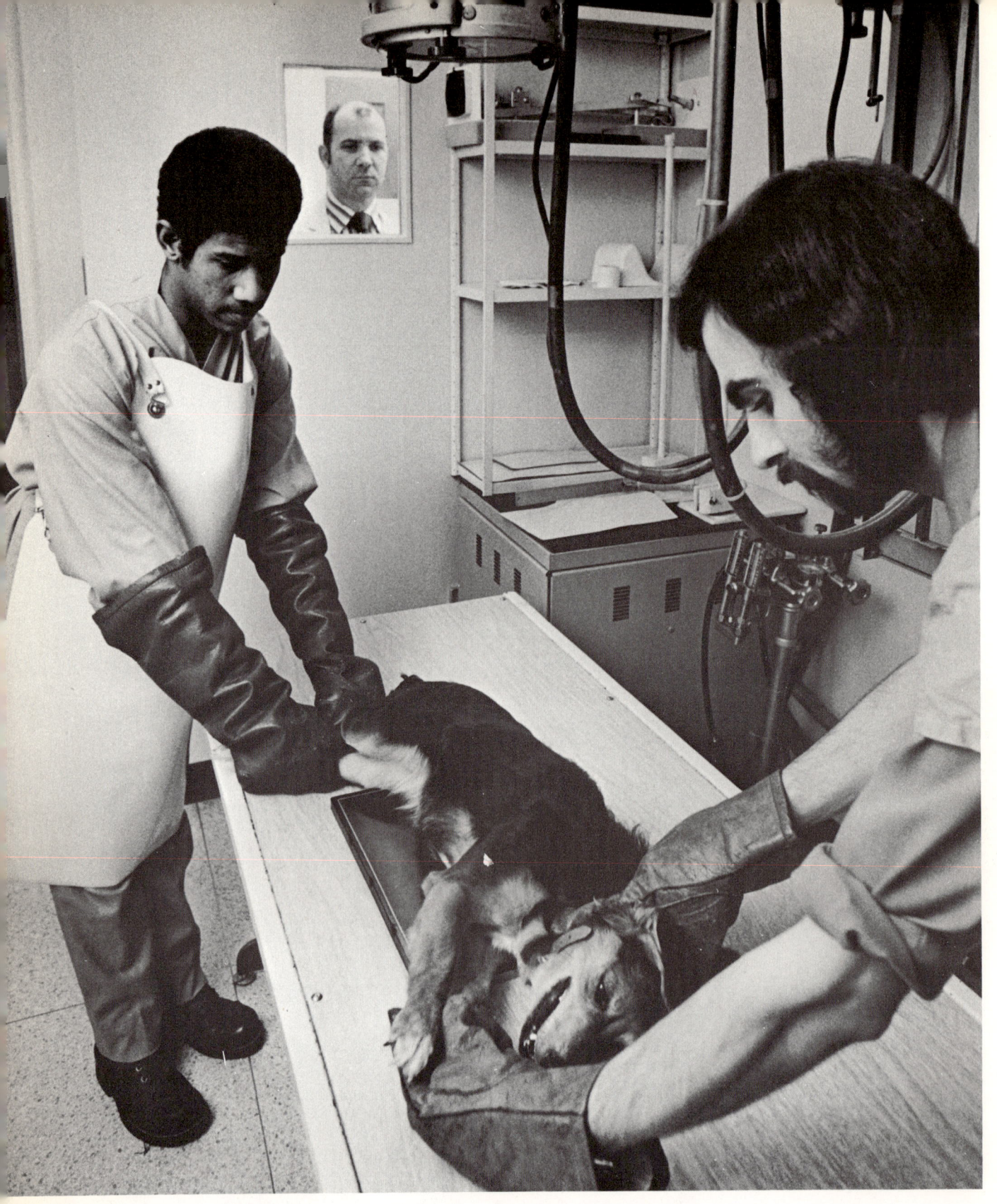

In the afternoon, Bambi was given some medical tests. Dr. Prasuhn wanted to make sure that he was right about Bambi's heart problem. John and another assistant, Herman George, held Bambi in place on the X-ray table. Dr. Stanley Harris, in the next room, pushed the camera button for X-ray pictures.

When the X rays were developed, Dr. Prasuhn and Dr. Harris had two clear pictures of Bambi's heart—one from the front, and the other from the side. By studying the pictures, the doctors could tell exactly where the problem was.

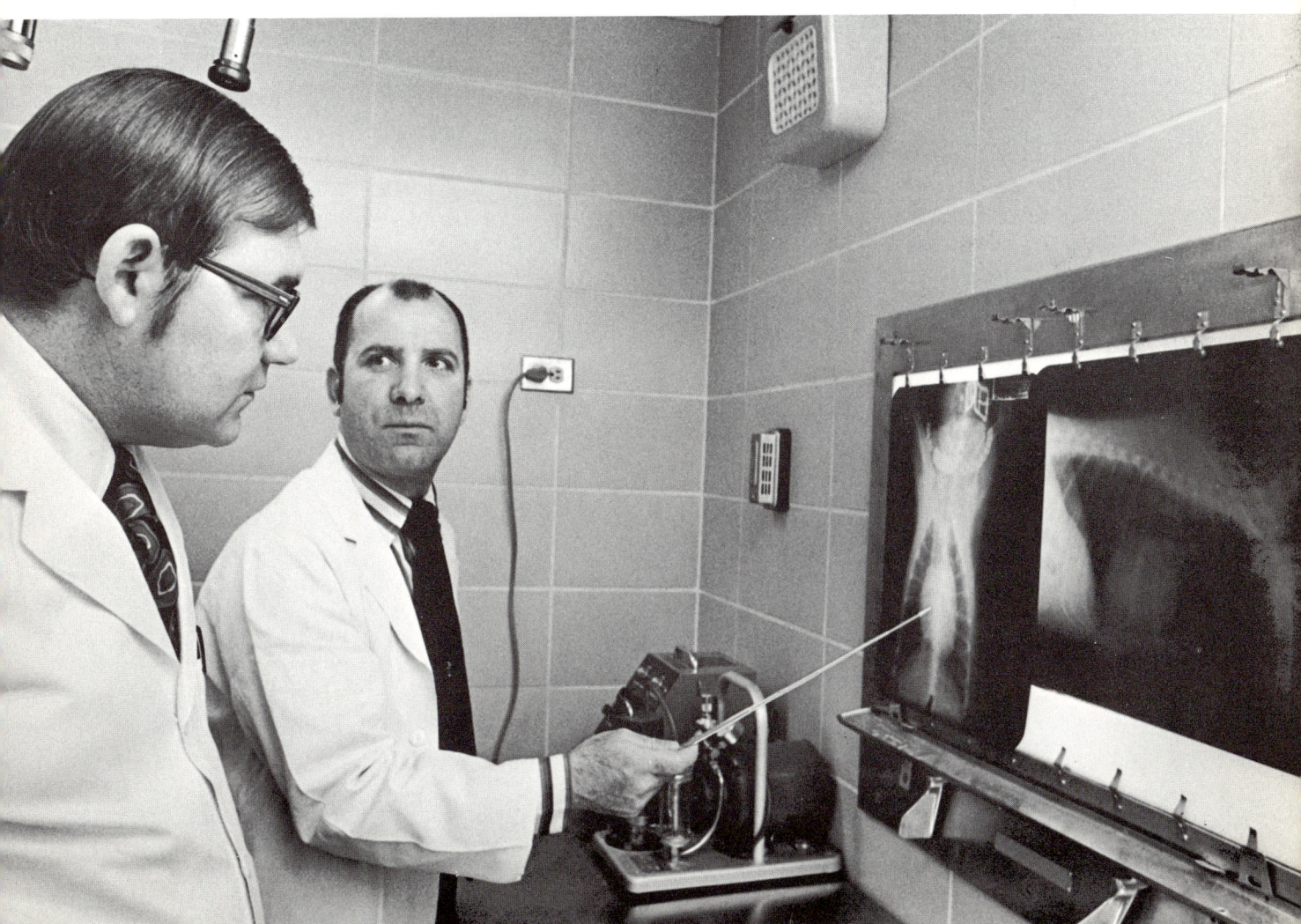

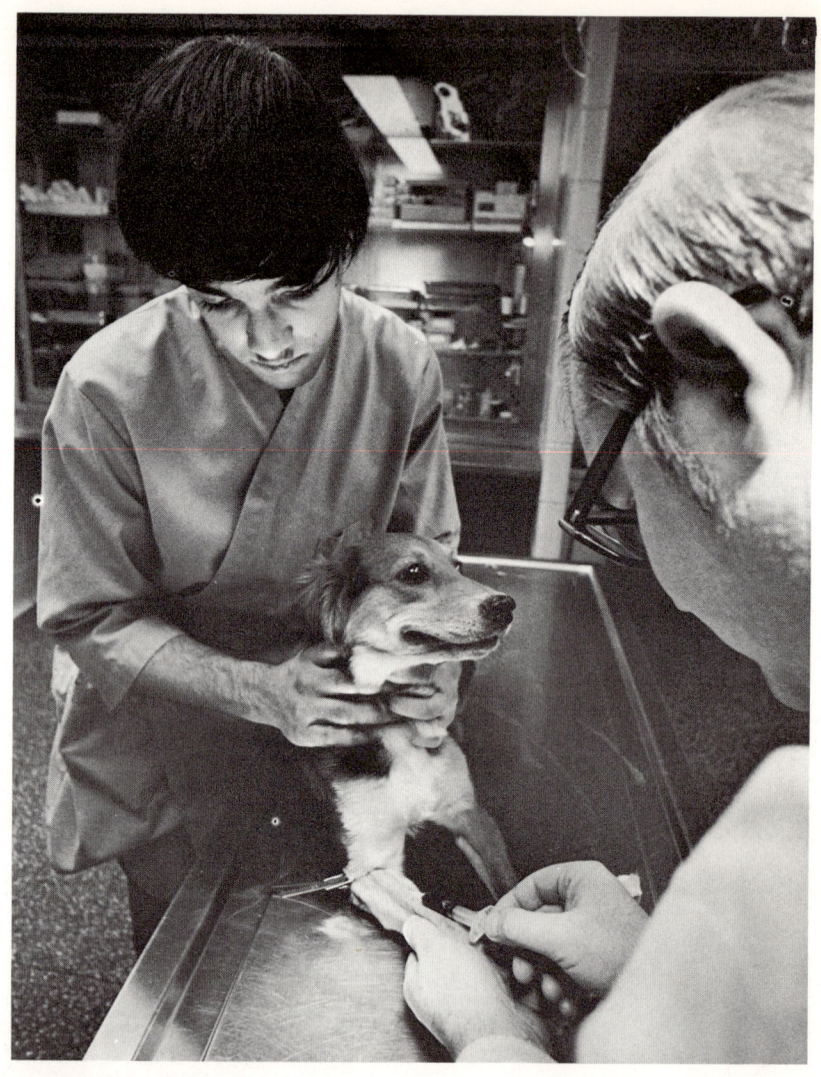

Next, Dr. Prasuhn drew some blood from Bambi's leg. To test the blood, he added some chemicals to the sample. Then, he put the sample on a *centrifuge*—a round tray that spins like a record player, only much faster. When the centrifuge stopped, the doctor looked at Bambi's blood sample under his microscope.

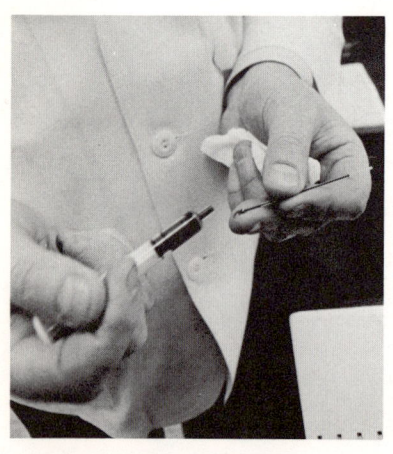 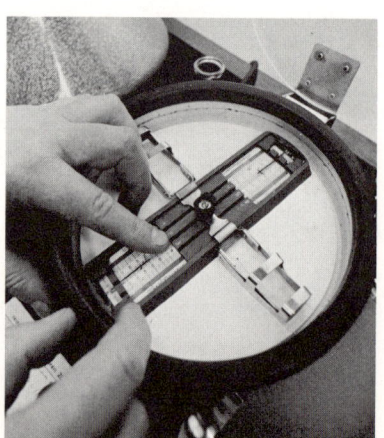 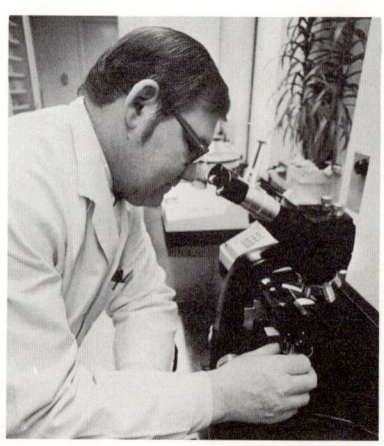

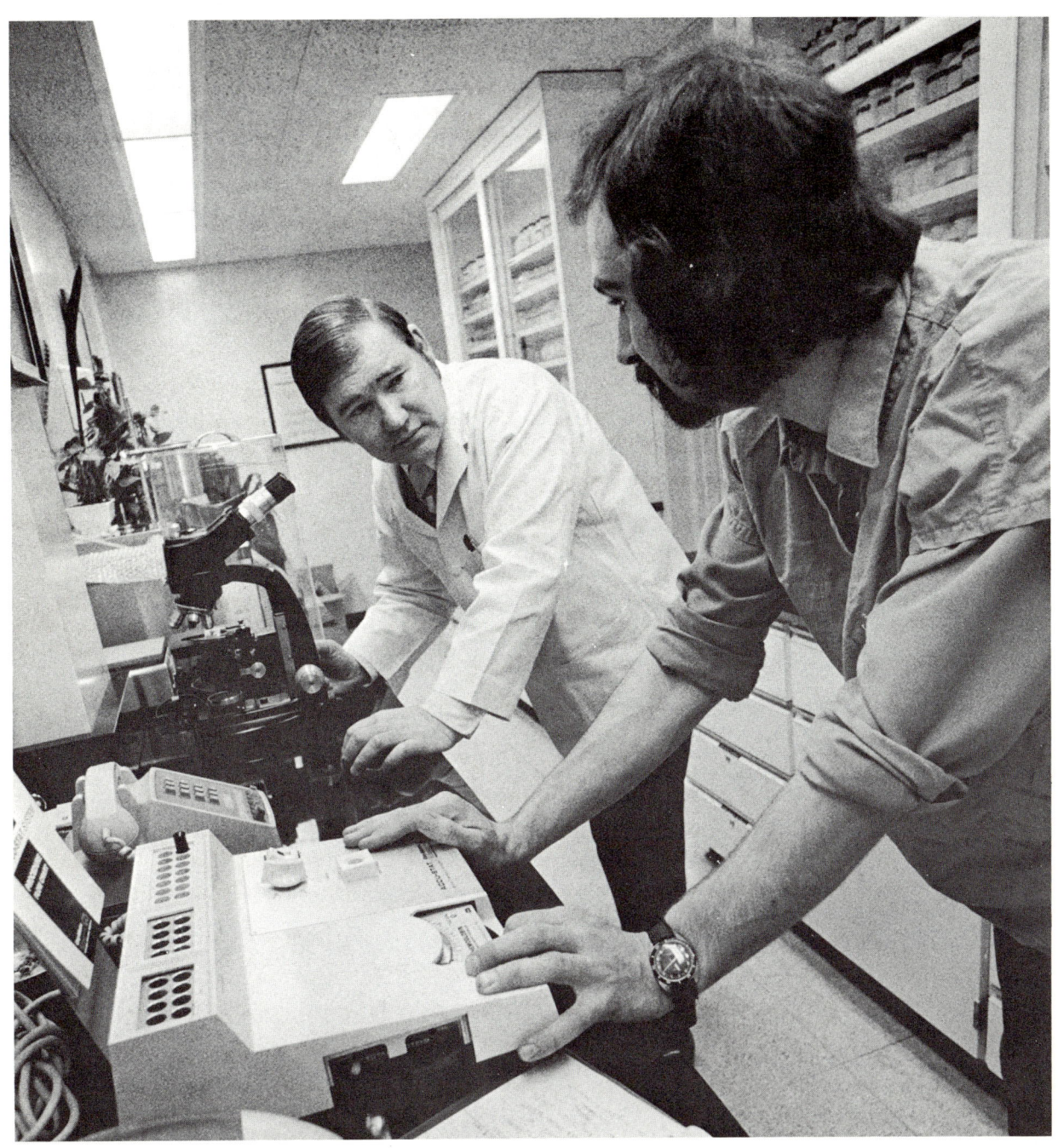

"Bambi's blood is normal," Dr. Prasuhn said to John. "That should help her to heal quickly after the operation. She'll have surgery first thing tomorrow morning."

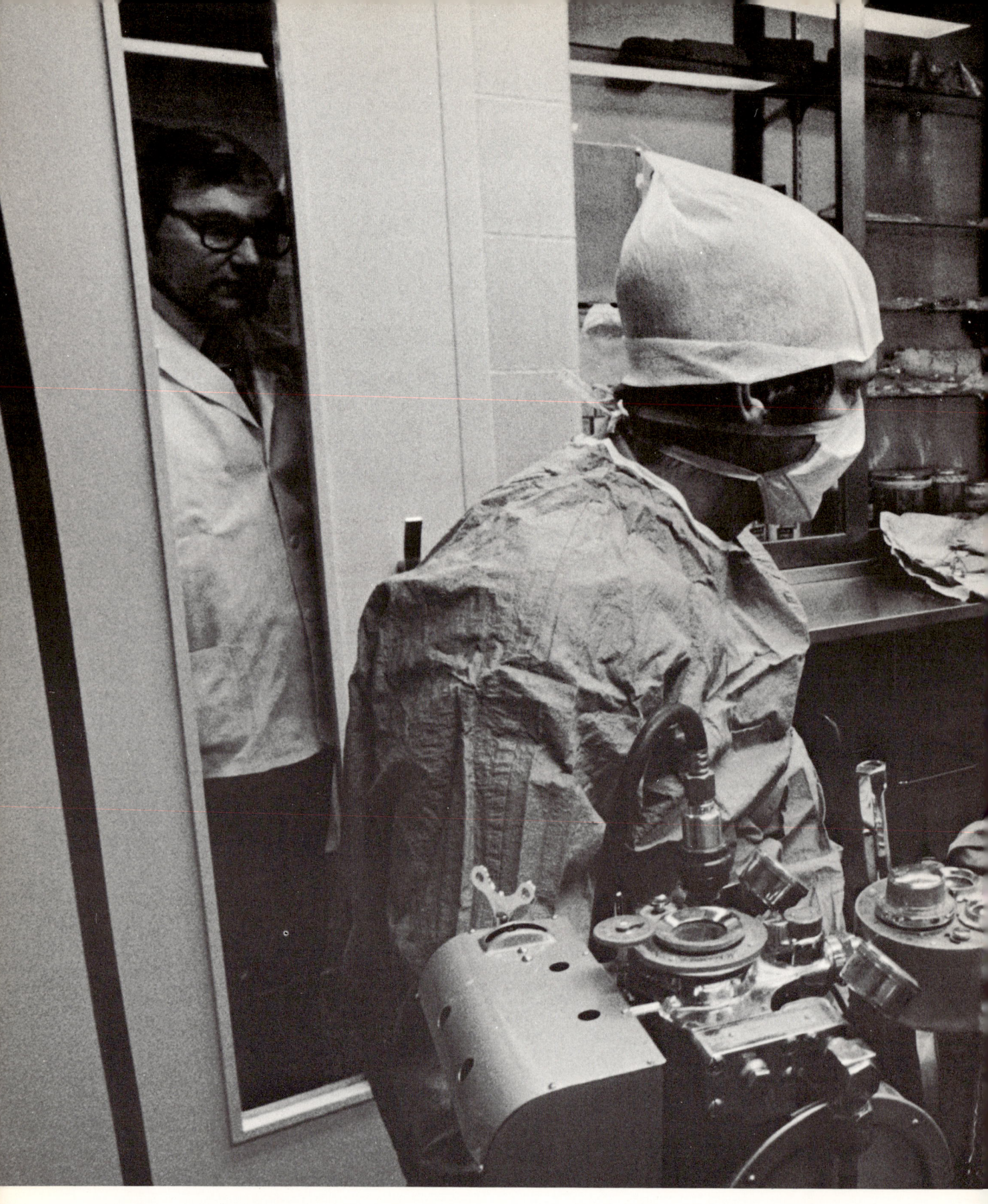

In the morning Dr. Prasuhn watched from outside the operating room as his surgical team worked on Bambi. The *anesthetist* was in charge of keeping Bambi asleep during the operation so she

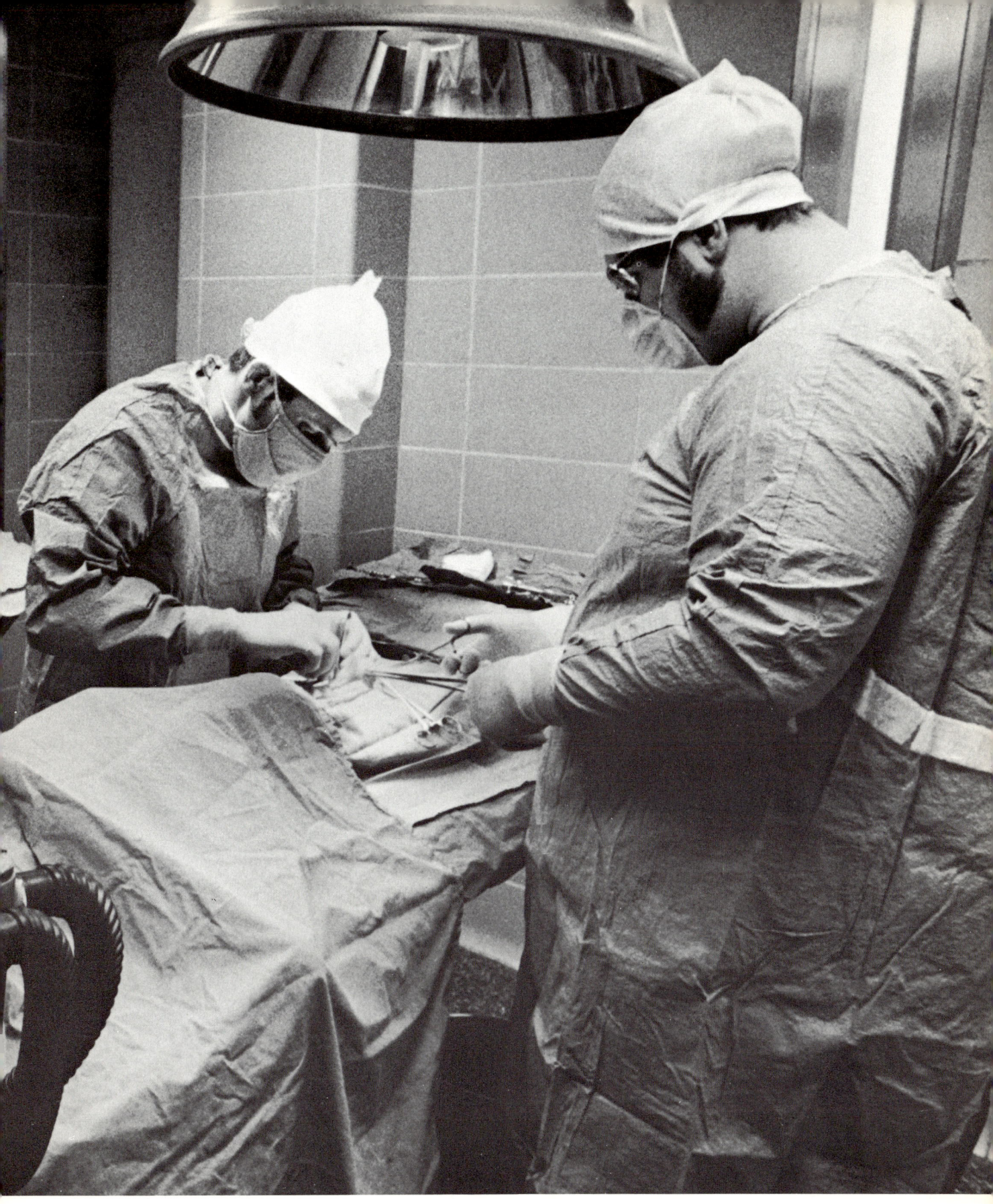

wouldn't feel any pain. Two *surgeons* opened up Bambi's chest, corrected the problem in her heart, and then sewed her up.

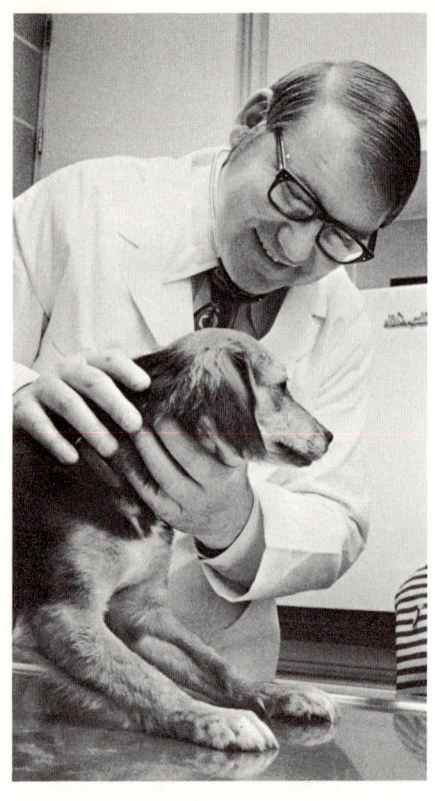

After a week had passed, Bambi had healed pretty well. She wasn't lazy anymore, her cough had disappeared, and she was a lot more interested in her food than she had been before the operation.

Dr. Prasuhn made some notes on Bambi's progress chart and then called the Reeds.

"Bambi's fine," he said. "Come and get her."

"Wheeee!" said Tony when he heard the good news.

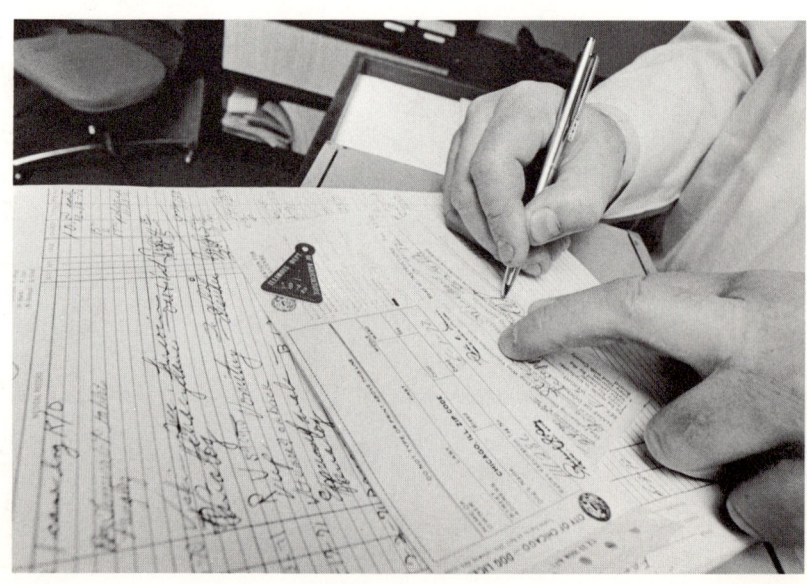

That evening, Dr. Prasuhn put some fresh bandages around Bambi's chest.

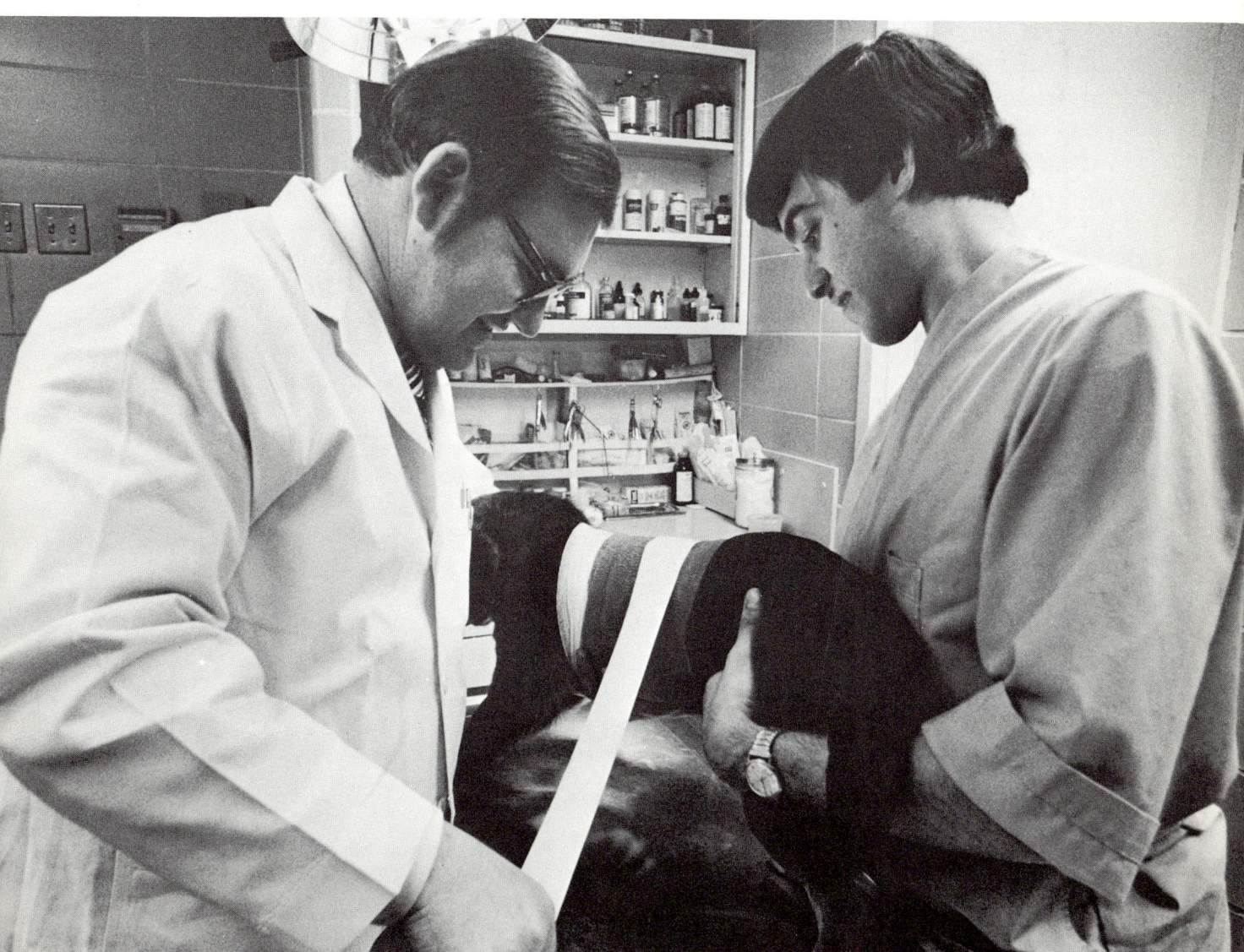

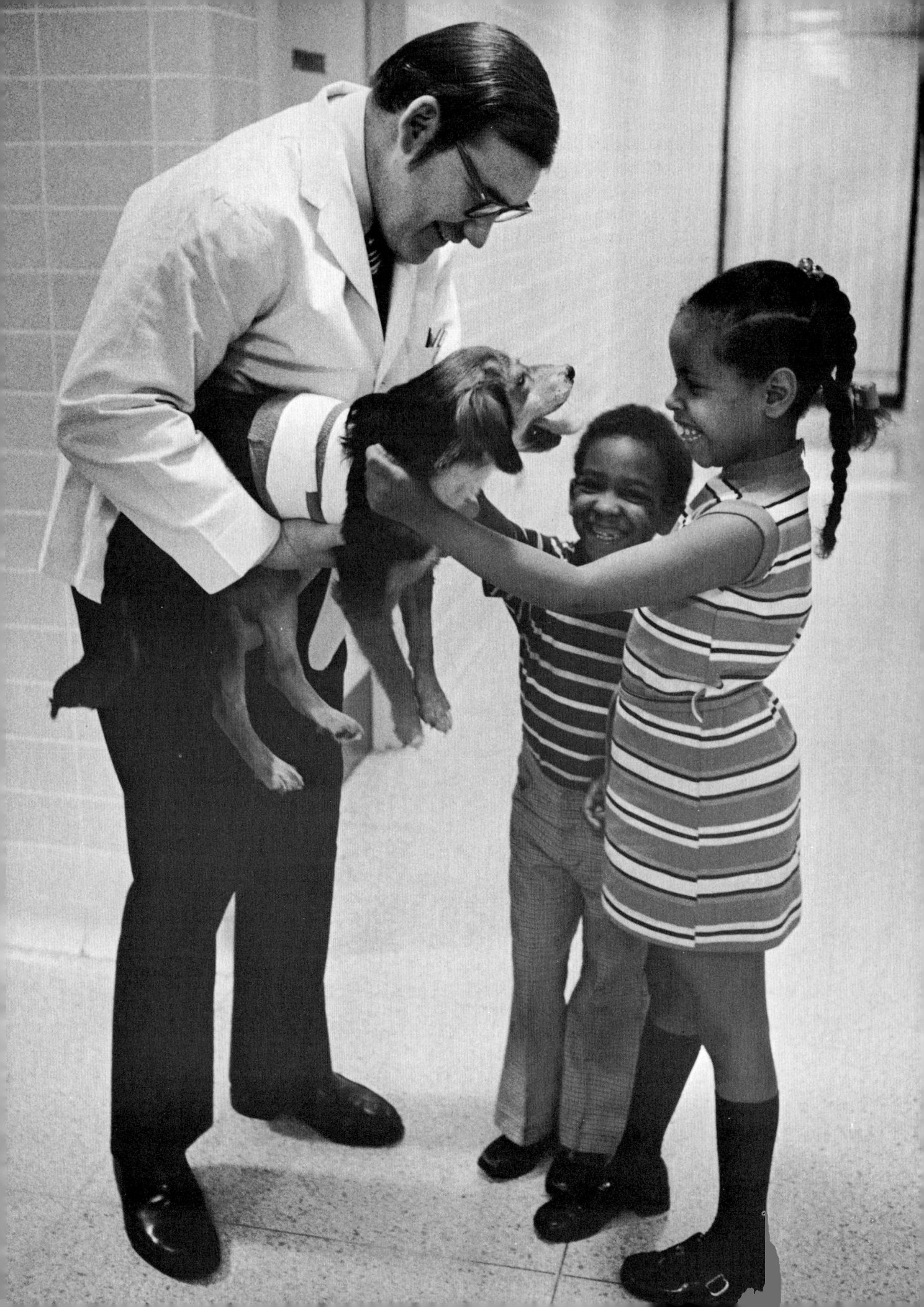

Then he carried Bambi into the corridor, where she yelped with joy to see her family again.

"Look how bright her eyes are," said Angie.

"She'll be able to walk around in about three days," said Dr. Prasuhn. "I'd like you to bring her in for a checkup in two weeks."

"May I take her to my ball game Saturday?" asked Tony.

"Of course you may," the doctor answered. "I told you she'd be as good as new. Actually, she'll be better than new because her heart is a lot stronger now."

"Thank you so much," said Ms. Reed to Dr. Prasuhn. "You've made our whole family happy."

"Look!" Angie giggled. "Even Bambi's smiling!"

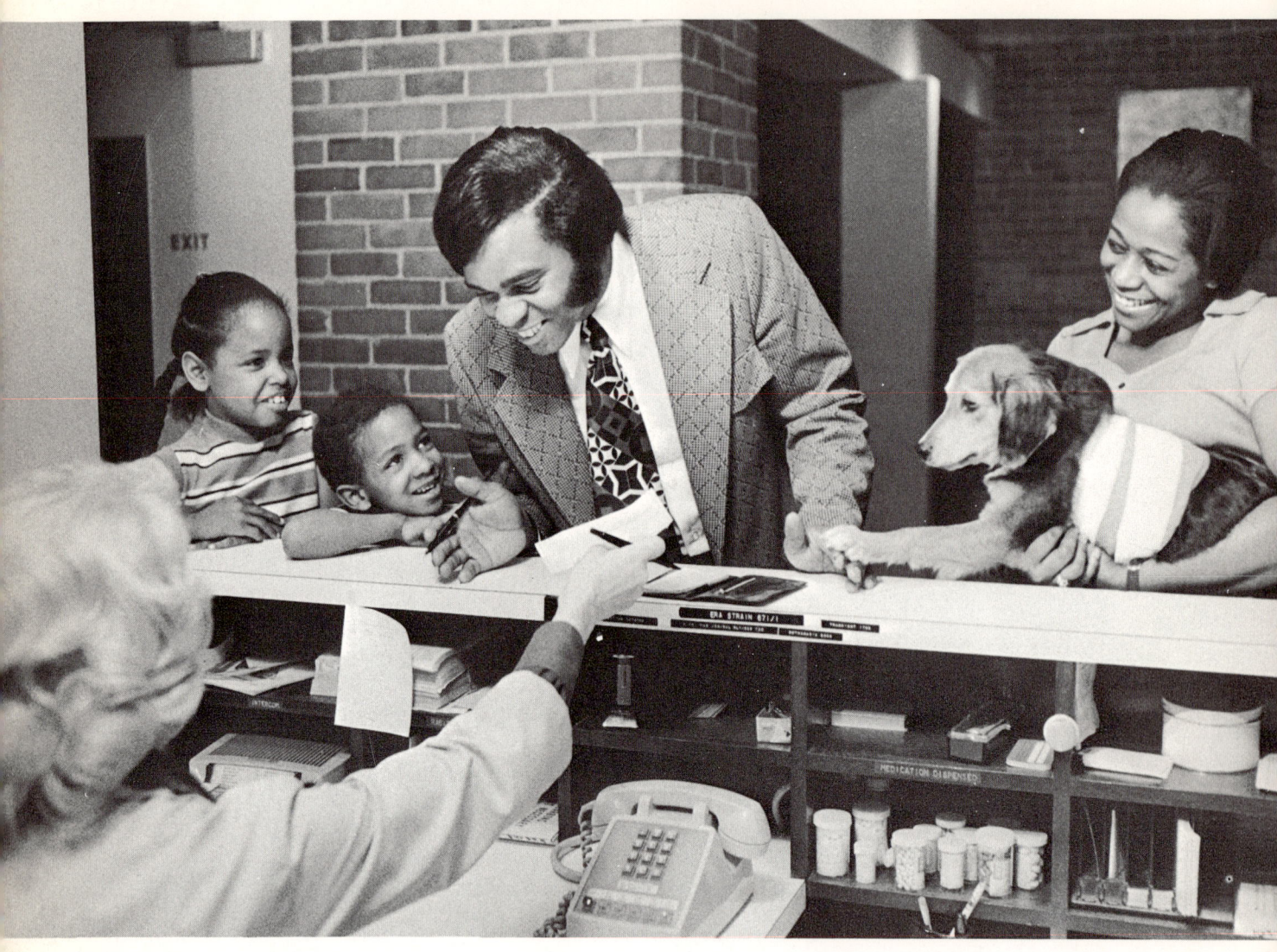

At the front desk, Mr. Reed wrote a check to pay for Bambi's operation. And in a few minutes the Reed family left the animal hospital and were on their way home.

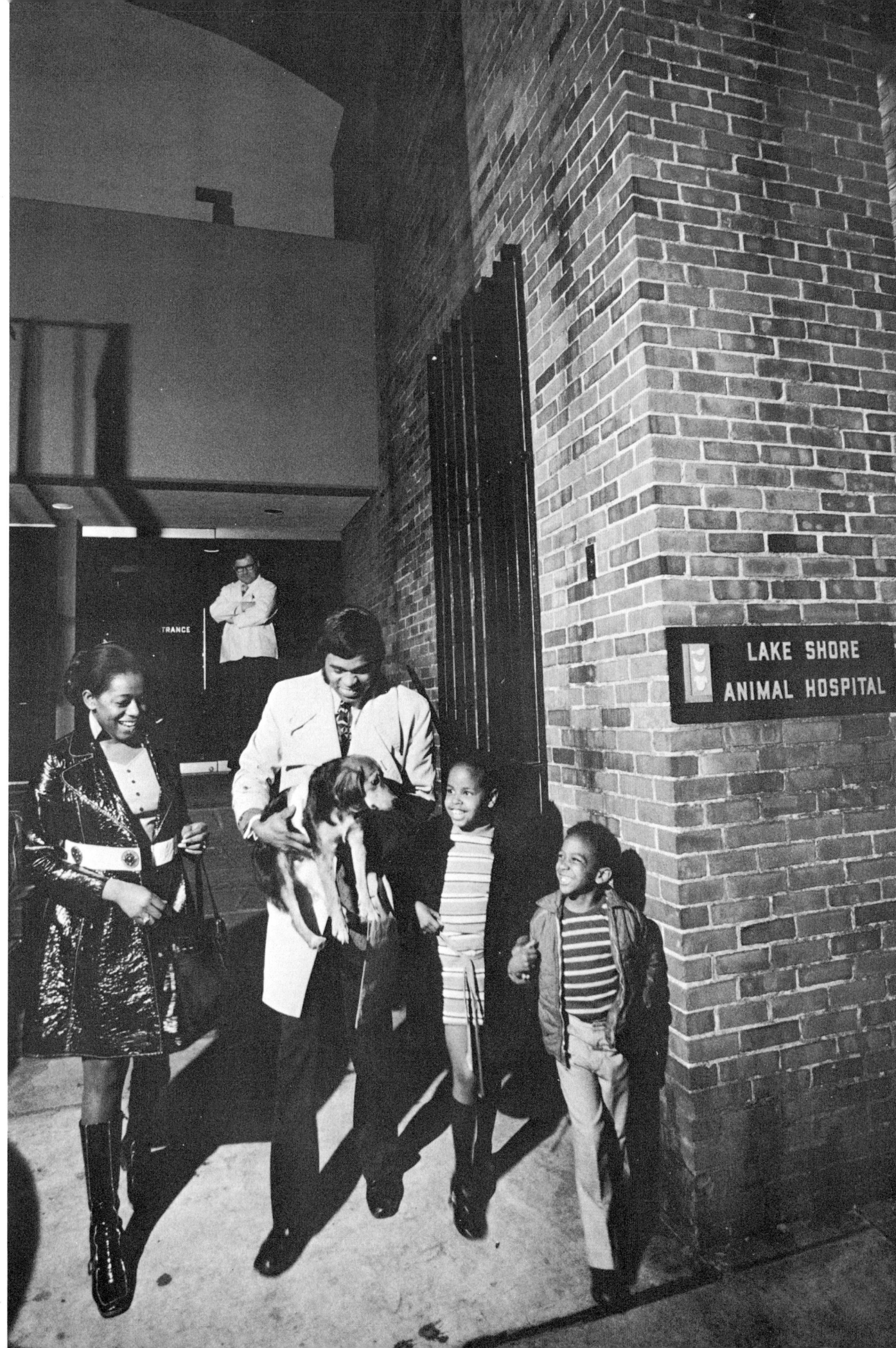

Other books by Arthur Shay:

What Happens at a Gas Station
What Happens at a Newspaper
What Happens at a Television Station
What Happens at the Circus
What Happens at the Library
What Happens at the Zoo
What Happens in a Car Factory
What Happens in a Skyscraper
What Happens When You Build a House
What Happens When You Go to the Hospital
What Happens When You Mail a Letter
What Happens When You Make a Telephone Call
What Happens When You Put Money in the Bank
What Happens When You Spend Money
What Happens When You Travel by Plane
What Happens When You Turn On the Light

What It's Like to Be a Dentist
What It's Like to Be a Doctor
What It's Like to Be a Fireman
What It's Like to Be a Musician
What It's Like to Be a Nurse
What It's Like to Be a Pilot
What It's Like to Be a Policeman
What It's Like to Be a Teacher